Beginner's Hack for CrossFit
"Workouts for Mental Toughness and Resilience".

Kevin N. Hise

Table of content

Chapter 1

Introduction

CrossFit exercises are noted for their intensity and ability to push participants to their physical limits. However, CrossFit is not just about the physical aspect of the workout. Mental toughness and resilience are equally vital to thrive in CrossFit. This is where our new booklet, "Beginner's Hack for CrossFit: Workouts for Mental Toughness and Resilience," comes in.

In this ebook, we will present an in-depth explanation of CrossFit routines and how they may be utilized to promote mental toughness and resilience. We will look into the significance of establishing mental toughness and resilience in CrossFit and how it may affect an individual's overall fitness and wellness.

Our objective and goal for this ebook are to equip newcomers with a complete guide on how to build mental toughness and resilience while practicing CrossFit exercises. We recognize that beginning a new fitness program may be scary, but we want to make the transition simpler by giving essential information and methods.

The next chapters will address numerous themes, including understanding mental toughness and resilience, CrossFit exercises for mental toughness and resilience, recovery tactics, establishing a resilient attitude, and a conclusion. We hope that after reading this booklet, you will have a better grasp of the significance of mental toughness and resilience in CrossFit and how to acquire it. Let's get started!

Chapter 2

Understanding Mental Toughness and Resilience

Mental toughness and resilience are crucial components for success in CrossFit. These two attributes are closely connected and work hand in hand to assist athletes accomplish their objectives. In this chapter, we will cover the concept of mental toughness, the characteristics of mentally tough individuals, the relevance of resilience in CrossFit, and tactics for improving mental toughness and resilience.

1. Definition of Mental Toughness:

Mental toughness may be characterized as the capacity to stay focused, motivated, and confident amid hard conditions. It requires the ability to push through physical and mental suffering, disappointments, and barriers without giving up or losing hope. Mental toughness is not something that comes naturally to everyone, but it may be acquired through training and practice.

2. Characteristics of Mentally Tough People:

Mentally strong individuals possess particular traits that enable them to navigate problems and conquer barriers. These include:

a. Resilience: Mentally strong people are resilient and can bounce back swiftly from setbacks and disappointments.

b. Perseverance: They have a strong sense of determination and are prepared to push through hard conditions.

c. Positive thinking: They have a positive mindset and believe in their abilities to conquer any difficulty.

d. Self-discipline: They have a great degree of self-discipline and can push themselves to their limits.

e. Focus: They can stay concentrated on their objectives, even when presented with distractions.

f. Adaptability: They can adjust to changing situations and are not readily sidetracked by unanticipated problems.

3. Importance of Resilience in CrossFit:

In CrossFit, resilience is crucial for success. Athletes that show resilience can push themselves to their limits, heal rapidly from injuries, and endure rigorous training. CrossFit exercises are meant to push competitors to their physical and mental limitations, and those who are not psychologically strong and resilient are likely to suffer.

Resilience is also crucial for injury prevention. Athletes who are psychologically robust and resilient are less prone to become disheartened by injuries and are more likely to bounce back fast. They are also more likely to take the required precautions to avoid future injuries, such as sufficient rest, diet, and rehabilitation.

4. Strategies for Developing Mental Toughness and Resilience:

Mental toughness and resilience are abilities that may be learned and enhanced through time. Here are some strategies to help build mental toughness and resilience:

a. Set objectives: Setting clear, measurable objectives is an excellent strategy to increase mental toughness and resilience. Goals offer athletes something to strive for and provide inspiration to keep pushing ahead.

b. Practice Visualization: Visualization is a strong practice that may help athletes gain mental toughness and resilience. Visualizing good outcomes may help athletes overcome self-doubt and remain motivated.

c. Embrace pain: In CrossFit, pain is unavoidable. Embracing pain and learning to push through it is a crucial element of establishing mental toughness and resilience.

d. Focus on the Process: Instead of concentrating entirely on the final result, athletes should focus on the process of obtaining their objectives. This entails breaking down big objectives into smaller, doable stages.

e. Learn from Failure: Failure is a normal part of the learning process. Mentally strong athletes learn from their setbacks and utilize them as chances to develop.

In conclusion, mental toughness and resilience are key to success in CrossFit. Developing these abilities takes time and practice, but with the correct mentality and tactics, anybody can become mentally robust and resilient. The following chapter will concentrate on particular CrossFit exercises that may assist improve mental toughness and resilience.

Chapter 3

CrossFit Workouts for Mental Toughness and Resilience

CrossFit is recognized for its rigorous and intensive exercises that push participants to their limits physically and emotionally. To effectively improve mental toughness and resilience in CrossFit, it is vital to integrate both physical and mental activities. In this chapter, we will explore numerous CrossFit exercises that are meant to not only enhance physical fitness but also create mental toughness and resilience.

1. "The Murph"
"The Murph" is a popular CrossFit exercise that was named after Lieutenant Michael Murphy, a Navy SEAL who was killed in action in Afghanistan. The exercise consists of:

- 1-mile run
- 100 pull-ups
- 200 push-ups
- 300 air squats
- 1-mile run

To properly test oneself psychologically, it is advised to conduct the exercise wearing a weighted vest. The exercise is not only physically hard but psychologically as well, pushing the athlete to push themselves despite the pain and tiredness.

2. "Fran"
"Fran" is a benchmark CrossFit exercise that comprises:

- 21 thrusters
- 21 pull-ups
- 15 thrusters
- 15 pull-ups

- 9 thrusters
- 9 pull-ups

The purpose of "Fran" is to finish the exercise as soon as possible, pushing oneself to the limit both physically and emotionally. The exercise demands a lot of mental courage to keep going despite the pain and tiredness.

3. "Fight Gone Bad"
"Fight Gone Bad" is another benchmark CrossFit session that consists of:

- 1 minute of wall balls
- 1 minute of sumo deadlift high-pulls
- 1 minute of box jumps
- 1 minute of push presses
- 1 minute of rowing for calories
- 1 minute of rest

The exercise is done three times, to earn the best overall score possible. The workout is meant to test people psychologically since they must keep pushing themselves through each minute of severe exertion.

4. "Kelly"
"Kelly" is a CrossFit exercise that consists of:

- 5 rounds for time:
- 400m run
- 30-box leaps
- 30 wall balls

The workout is meant to be physically and intellectually tough, pushing users to push themselves through each set of exercises.

5. "Grace"
"Grace" is a CrossFit exercise that consists of:

- 30 clean and jerks for timing

The workout is supposed to be finished as rapidly as possible, with participants pushing themselves mentally to execute the activity as effectively as feasible.

Tips for Completing the Workouts Successfully:

To properly finish these CrossFit exercises, it is crucial to concentrate on appropriate form and technique, as well as pace oneself. It is also crucial to keep mentally engaged and motivated, pushing oneself through the pain and tiredness.

Modifications for Beginners:

For novices, it is advisable to start with lesser weights and fewer repetitions to build up strength and endurance gradually. It is also crucial to concentrate on good form and technique to prevent damage. Additionally, modifications such as assisted pull-ups or box jumps can be made to accommodate individual fitness levels.

Overall, these CrossFit routines are meant to not only enhance physical fitness but also create mental toughness and resilience. By mixing physical and mental training, athletes may push themselves to their limits and gain the mental power required to conquer any hurdle in CrossFit and life.

Chapter 4

Recovery Strategies for Mental Toughness and Resilience

A. Explanation of the Importance of Recovery for Mental Toughness and Resilience

When it comes to growing mental toughness and resilience, recuperation is just as crucial as the exercises themselves. Recovery is the act of enabling the body and mind to relax and heal after a difficult exercise, and it's crucial for avoiding burnout and injury.

In CrossFit, recovery is essential for building mental toughness and resilience. By taking the time to recuperate correctly, athletes may minimize their chance of injury, enhance their performance, and acquire the mental and emotional fortitude required to handle even the most grueling exercises.

B. Strategies for Recovery after Mentally Challenging Workouts

1. Nutrition

Nutrition is a critical element of rehabilitation since it supplies the body with the nutrition and energy it needs to repair and rebuild muscle tissue. After a psychologically difficult exercise, it's vital to replenish with a balance of protein and carbs. Some excellent alternatives include:

- Lean proteins like chicken, fish, and tofu
- Complex carbs like sweet potatoes, quinoa, and brown rice

- Fruits and vegetables for vitamins and minerals

In addition to solid meals, athletes may want to explore taking protein drinks or other supplements to assist them in their recuperation.

2. Sleep

Sleep is another crucial element of rehabilitation, as it helps the body and mind to relax and replenish. After a psychologically taxing exercise, it's crucial to prioritize sleep to allow the body adequate time to recuperate.

Most individuals require between seven and nine hours of sleep every night, but athletes may need even more. To increase sleep quality, athletes may try:

- Establishing a consistent sleep pattern

- Creating a calm nighttime routine
- Avoiding devices and bright lights before sleep
- Keeping the bedroom cold and dark

3. Self-Care

Self-care is any action that promotes relaxation, stress alleviation, and general well-being. After a cognitively tough exercise, it's crucial to emphasize self-care to assist the body and mind recuperate. Some examples of self-care activities include:

- Yoga or stretching
- Meditation or deep breathing
- Massage or foam rolling
- Taking a hot bath or shower
- Spending time in nature

C. Importance of Recovery for Injury Prevention

Finally, it's important to note that recovery is critical for injury prevention. Without adequate recuperation, athletes may endure burnout, tiredness, and even injury. By taking the time to rest and recuperate, athletes may lower their risk of injury and remain psychologically strong and resilient over the long term.

In addition to the healing measures outlined above, athletes should also listen to their bodies and take rest days as required. It's vital to remember that mental toughness and resilience aren't formed overnight - they're the consequence of constant, concentrated work over time. By prioritizing recuperation, athletes may remain on track with their training and continue to make progress toward their objectives.

Chapter 5
Building a Resilient Mindset

A. Importance of mentality in CrossFit

CrossFit is more than simply a physical workout; it is an attitude. It needs a strong attitude to push through the hard exercises, overcome mental blockages, and remain devoted to attaining fitness objectives. A resilient mentality is crucial to success in CrossFit and may help athletes handle the ups and downs of training.

B. Strategies for creating a resilient mentality

1. Positive self-talk
Positive self-talk is an excellent technique to cultivate a resilient attitude. It includes replacing negative ideas with

positive affirmations. For example, instead of stating "I can't do this," you may say "I am capable of achieving this." Positive self-talk helps to boost confidence, enhance motivation, and decrease stress.

2. Visualization

Visualization is a strong technique for improving mental toughness and resilience. It entails constructing mental representations of reaching your objectives. For example, envisioning oneself finishing a challenging exercise successfully might help you generate confidence and drive. Visualization helps to increase mental toughness by helping people to concentrate on the good parts of their performance and overcome negative ideas.

3. Goal setting

Goal setting is a crucial element of creating a resilient attitude. It entails creating specified, measurable, attainable, relevant, and time-bound (SMART) objectives. Setting realistic objectives helps people to remain motivated, focused, and devoted to their training. Achieving little objectives may create a feeling of satisfaction and develop confidence.

4. Mindfulness
Mindfulness is the discipline of being present in the moment and focusing on the current experience. It enables people to become more conscious of their thoughts and feelings and to adopt a non-judgmental attitude towards them. Mindfulness may assist people to manage stress, increase their mental concentration, and develop resilience.

C. Importance of mentality in daily life

A resilient attitude is not just vital in CrossFit, but also in daily life. It may enable people to overcome problems, manage stress, and accomplish their objectives. By creating a resilient mentality via positive self-talk, visualization, goal planning, and mindfulness, people may enhance their mental toughness, minimize negative thoughts, and boost their overall well-being.

Conclusion

Building a resilient mentality is a vital component of success in CrossFit. By developing positive self-talk, visualization, goal setting, and mindfulness, individuals can build mental toughness and resilience, which will help them to push through challenging workouts, overcome mental blocks, and achieve their fitness goals. A

resilient attitude is not only vital in CrossFit but also in daily life, since it may allow people to overcome
problems, handle stress, and attain their objectives.

Chapter 6

Conclusion

Congratulations, you have made it to the conclusion of this ebook! By now, you should have a strong idea of the significance of mental toughness and resilience in CrossFit, as well as some successful exercises and tactics to help you improve these abilities.

In this last chapter, we will summarize everything we have learned and provide some closing comments and encouragement for readers.

Recap on the Importance of Mental Toughness and Resilience in CrossFit

As we mentioned in prior chapters, mental toughness, and resilience are crucial attributes for success in CrossFit.

These abilities help athletes to push through physical pain, overcome mental hurdles, and remain motivated in the face of adversity.

We discussed the notion of mental toughness, which incorporates attributes like tenacity, drive, and the capacity to remain focused on objectives. We also looked at the role of resilience in CrossFit, which helps athletes to bounce back from losses, learn from errors, and remain devoted to their training.

Recap of the CrossFit Workouts and Strategies for Building Mental Toughness and Resilience

In Chapter 3, we reviewed many CrossFit routines that are especially good for strengthening mental toughness and resilience. These included "The Murph," "Fran," "Fight Gone Bad," "Kelly," and

"Grace." We also provided tips for completing these workouts successfully and modifications for beginners.

In Chapter 4, we addressed the role of recuperation in mental toughness and resilience. We gave suggestions for recovery following psychologically taxing exercises, including diet, sleep, and self-care and underlined the relevance of recovery in injury prevention.

In Chapter 5, we focused on establishing a resilient attitude. We explored the significance of attitude in CrossFit and daily life and presented tools for establishing a resilient mindset, including positive self-talk, visualization, goal planning, and mindfulness.

Final Thoughts and Encouragement

We hope that this booklet has been useful in giving you the skills you need to build mental toughness and resilience in your CrossFit training. Remember, these traits take time and work to acquire, so don't be disheartened if you don't see results right away.

With constant practice and a desire to go beyond your comfort zone, you can establish a resilient attitude and acquire the mental fortitude essential to thrive in CrossFit and life. So get out there, take on those difficult exercises, and never give up on your ambitions. You've got this!